Table of Contents

8.1. Advancements in Surgical Techniques

8.2. Clinical Trials and Future Directions

Understanding the Purpose and Side Effects of Brain Aneurysm Clipping Surgery

1. Introduction to Brain Aneurysms

The occurrence of brain aneurysms can occur at any age or at any time, but the routine check-up may not detect them in many young and during some particular periods. In the United States, the patient used to know of people who have unruptured brain aneurysm, over 2 million people, according to data from the Brain Aneurysms Foundation. Silverstein and the reported team found with the accumulation or genetics on blood congestion or high blood pressure that made the blood vessels of the aneurysms swell, they said according to findings published in the journal Nature Genetics. Usually, brain aneurysms can be treated before they burst by trained neurosurgeons. Even though these blood vessels may be taken care of after the rupture, the beliefs of the patient were uncertain, and it may affect the mood.

Brain aneurysm generally refers to the dilatation or ballooning of arteries' walls, which are small and large tubes that help transport oxygenated blood to various parts of the brain. Protective layers of the arteries can weaken the wall and a brain aneurysm is formed. The pressure lands on the weak area, and a bulge of sorts is formed with weakening walls. The brain aneurysms are harmful because they can burst easily and cause bleeding in the brain, which can lead to increased intracranial pressure and death. Brain aneurysms cause strokes, heart attacks, brain damage, and death, and the complications can cause different after-effects based on severity.

2. Overview of Brain Aneurysm Clipping Surgery

What are the limitations of clipping? It is important to note that once the aneurysm is secured by a clip, it is usually considered cured. However, occasionally an aneurysm can begin to regrow at the neck of the aneurysm, which may require additional treatment such as coiling of the aneurysm. Some aneurysms may not be treatable by clipping. In these cases, aneurysm coiling is often possible. However, in some cases, the aneurysm may not be treatable by a minimally invasive approach, and treatment may involve a craniotomy with clipping of the aneurysm, either alone or in combination with endovascular coiling.

Clipping procedure. The most common way to clip a brain aneurysm is from the outside of the skull. In this procedure, the surgeon makes an opening in the skull called a craniotomy. After making the opening in the skull, the surgeon spreads the brain tissue apart to locate the aneurysm. Once the aneurysm is located, the surgeon will place a small metal clip on the neck of the aneurysm to reduce the blood flow into it. Then the skull will be closed with metal plates and screws. The bone flap is usually put back at the end of the procedure, unless there is a medical reason to leave it out.

Surgery can be used to treat brain aneurysms, which are balloon-like bulges that form in the wall of a blood vessel. Brain aneurysm clipping is a surgical procedure in which a metal clip is placed in the brain to try to prevent the aneurysm from bleeding or from growing larger.

2.1. Definition and Procedure

Prior to your brain aneurysm clipping surgery, an intravenous (IV) line will be inserted into your arm or hand by the anesthesiologist. You'll be placed under general anesthesia, and the surgical team will shave some hair from your head and sterilize the area that will be operated on. Brain aneurysm clipping surgery can be performed in various ways. Most often, it is performed through a craniotomy, in which a surgical cut is made in the scalp. A piece of the skull bone or bones is removed to access the aneurysm. Although clipping is performed at this time, additional surgeries may be needed, such as for placing a ventricular drain to allow the drainage of cerebrospinal fluid (CSF). In the neurointerventional angiography suite, it is possible to undergo a less invasive procedure with a similar purpose called the balloon test occlusion or BTO. In the BTO procedure, a catheter is navigated into the arteries where it can block blood flow to the aneurysm. If the patient's neurological condition does not deteriorate, the artery can be blocked with a coil or glue. Finally, even if open surgery is the initial plan, endovascular coiling might be performed if a craniotomy with clipping is attempted without success due to an aneurysm's location, shape, and other characteristics.

Brain aneurysm clipping surgery, or "surgical clipping," is a procedure most often performed following a ruptured aneurysm. An aneurysm is a blood vessel in the brain that bulges out, like a bubble. If that bubble bursts, it can result in a brain hemorrhage and put an individual's life at risk.

That is one of the key reasons brain aneurysm clipping surgery is recommended. Clipping surgery is most often performed going through the skull or cranium in conjunction with a craniotomy, although minimally invasive techniques are developing, including insertion through the leg in an angiography suite.

3. Purpose of Brain Aneurysm Clipping Surgery

Neurosurgeons use brain aneurysm clipping surgery to repair the aneurysm if it is either in a longer, larger, or irregularly-shaped artery, which might predispose the patient to the aneurysm coming back with endovascular procedures, a partially calcified and/or a large aneurysm, as the clip might have more staying power than endovascular coils in such aneurysms as a primary procedure. This list of criteria for treating the aneurysm with aneurysm clipping surgery is likely not complete. It's important that you discuss your condition with a qualified doctor who can help you understand the treatment options that may be available to you. Over time, brain aneurysm repair with clipping can achieve the same reliably excellent long-term outcome as coiling. That means that the patient can live just as long as he or she would have with the brain aneurysm if it hadn't ruptured, be just as intelligent, and be just as likely to return to their pre-ruptured state, as a patient who had coiling. The chief benefit of clipping a brain aneurysm instead of coiling is that the chance of the aneurysm's coming back after clipping is either stable or somewhat less, depending on the size and shape of the aneurysm in question. Explains brain aneurysm repair options.

Brain aneurysm clipping surgery is a surgical procedure used to treat an aneurysm, which is a ballooning of an artery in the brain. The purpose of aneurysm clipping surgery is to seal off the aneurysm from blood flow in order to prevent potential life-threatening bleeding. The aneurysm will likely be repaired with a clip, to cut off blood flow to and from the bulge. The clip is made of a non-rusting material such as titanium, and it is left inside the cranium. To reach the aneurysm, the neurosurgeon moves the brain tissue (as gently as possible) to perform the repair. Brain aneurysm clipping surgery is a whole-brain surgery and patients are put to sleep using general anesthesia.

3.1. Prevention of Rupture

Technically successful aneurysm surgical treatment prevents aneurysm ruptures, and after surgery, the risk of subarachnoid hemorrhage and perioperative risks are gone. After surgical clipping, aneurysms thrombose gradually, and healing of tissue at the aneurysm neck and in the clips takes place. Because this process starts immediately after aneurysm clipping, the risk for rupture due to aneurysm growth or recanalization of the aneurysm cavity as might be seen in long-term follow-up after endovascular coiling is effectively eliminated within short time. However, the intraoperative aneurysm rupture creates conditions similar to a spontaneous rupture; therefore, the previously discussed pathophysiological cascades are comparable for surgically and conservatively managed SAH.

One of the main purposes of microsurgical intervention to obliterate a brain aneurysm is to eliminate the risks of rupture. It is particularly important for cerebral aneurysms because the resulting blood flow from progressive aneurysm rupture can rapidly cause catastrophic life-threatening clinical conditions. These typically are a result of hydrocephalus, brain edema, or brain infarction. Moreover, aneurysmal hemorrhage caused by rupture continues to have high morbidity and mortality. Because a ruptured aneurysm could carry the immense risks of subsequent disability and death, preventing rupture by microsurgical obliteration of the aneurysm is often recommended for high-risk patients.

4. Risk Factors for Brain Aneurysm Formation

Regardless, taking caffeine and nicotine does not increase the risk of developing brain aneurysms. It results in the fact that the risk of a brain aneurysm becoming empty, in particular, patients who are older than 60 might have frequency forecasts if they are in the range of developing aneurysms of various sizes during their lifetimes. It can be understood from this report that 27% of females, 29% of men, and three out of every hundred women above 60 have some sort of individual's brain aneurysm. Only about 2 percent, which is 2% to 3 out of 100, of brain aneurysms ever burst. Executing the required risks to manage an unruptured aneurysm, therefore, would be more dangerous than the life-long hemorrhage possibility. Blood from a broken aneurysm passes into the space around the brain, part towards the brain, and part towards the mind.

Brain aneurysm formation takes place due to the weakening of the arterial wall. This may happen because of a specific group of risk factors. Diseases or problems that are linked to strengthening the walls of blood vessels within the brain are generally believed to be risks for brain aneurysm formation. Brain aneurysms are not the cause of constant headaches. Aneurysms may be there due to diseases such as arteriosclerosis and certain diseases present at birth. Another risk factor that is considered to reveal the probability of brain aneurysm creation is hereditary; if the first-degree member of the family has a brain aneurysm, then the percentage of additional members to have brain aneurysm increases beyond the general population's 2 percent. There appears to be a definite mind aneurysm's run; however, it happens that it occurs as a result of an identical environmental condition in addition to the inherited trait.

4.1. Genetic Predisposition

Lollipop-shaped aneurysms seem to have hereditary features and it has been suggested that they could be associated with the development of the disease. Brain aneurysms tend to cluster in families, partially due to shared environments and partially inherited traits. Therefore, individuals with a first-degree relative who has an aneurysm are approximately three times more likely to develop an aneurysm themselves than the general population. Further genetic investigations need to be conducted to reveal the pathways affected by the presence of IL-1β, -2, -4, -8, -10, -L, TNF-α, and TGF-β in order to provide new perspectives on the treatment of brain aneurysms. In our future studies, we are planning to include these aforementioned possible genetic defect tests. We have identified various environmental and genetic risk factors as a result of a thorough analysis of our series. Due to the fact that individuals with this genetic or family predisposition are born with and develop brain aneurysms, we believe that further research in this field of disease will contribute to understanding more fully the nature of genetic and environmental lesions for the disease.

Although the pathogenesis of brain aneurysm still remains obscure, a significant amount of studies have dealt with possible risk factors for the development of the disease. This retrospective analysis further led us to present a number of genetic predisposition risk factors for brain aneurysm formation.

5. Common Side Effects of Brain Aneurysm Clipping Surgery

There are several frequent side effects of brain aneurysm clipping that occur after surgery. Ruptured or unruptured aneurysms in the brain can cause the following symptoms: frequently feeling weary, having problems with your cognition or conduct, having difficulties in communication or speech, having weak or paralyzed muscles, having headaches, seizures, vision issues. Pressure on nerve centers in the brain can cause nerve-connected signs or symptoms. The most popular artery that supplies blood to the brain and conveys signals from this first layer to deeper fillings is the anterior connecting artery. When ruptured, an aneurysm can harm the brain and generate lengthy mental harm. Configuration An aneurysm that is about to rupture or has recently ruptured can be adjusted using a process called aneurysm clipping. An aneurysm may be caused by a weak area that swells off. This further weakens the artery wall and causes a balloon to swell.

Brain aneurysm clipping surgery is a protective procedure that reduces an individual's risk of life-threatening bleeding and rebleeding from an aneurysm, or balloon trip, in a blood vessel in the brain tissue. Before having this type of surgery, you should be aware of the possible side effects and the reasons why they happen.

5.1. Infection and Bleeding

Bleeding may occur both during and after the operation, causing bruising. A bruise or hematoma develops when the blood released from the operation coagulates. The hematoma can become too big and put pressure on the bone, all the surrounding tissue, and the nerves. Surgical trauma and duration, craniotomy (cranium opening), and qualities around the cerebrum may influence the incidence of hematomas. This can irritate the brain and cause the baby to face more challenges and have a longer recovery period. To avoid bleeding, the neurosurgeon will work carefully. When designing the features of the brain aneurysm, a microsurgical approach demands a minimum damage to the core.

Bleeding

Infection can be a serious matter, and development of an infection at the surgical site or in the skull is frequently associated with the bone becoming infected (osteomyelitis). Severe infections can lead to serious illness, permanent health problems, and an inability to complete recovery. Sterility is maintained during every neurosurgery. The face, skull, and heart will be washed and handled wisely as a result of this. The contaminated bandage will be removed from the neurosurgeon in order to guarantee that it does not unintentionally get rid of any illness on the bandage. They typically utilize Teflon-coated sutures to help avoid infection. Following surgery, certain medications ought to be given in order to reduce the possibility of infection. If an infection exists, antibiotics or other therapies may be required.

Infection

6. Recovery and Rehabilitation After Surgery

Cognitive and speech therapy that will focus more specifically on the thinking and speech aspects of the brain that a stroke hits are also important. This therapy can be one-on-one with a therapist or through group therapy sessions. Following inpatient rehab, occasional outpatient therapy may be ordered. Less frequently, some survivors of large or very severe strokes require longer-term or even lifelong inpatient assisted living or nursing care. The overall course is highly variable based on the size and location of the stroke, age of the patient, and their pre-stroke health and support system. Many people develop complications that can slow or otherwise complicate the recovery process, such as urinary tract infections, skin breakdown, and blood clots in the leg. These conditions also need to be addressed by their care professional. Most strokes require at least 6 months to a year for substantial recovery, though some strokes more severe than a brain aneurysm bleed may never markedly improve.

Recovering from brain aneurysm surgery requires physicians at the hospital to monitor you closely for complications. For instance, they will monitor you for any signs of stroke, infection, or changes in consciousness for weeks after the surgery. Once the patient leaves the hospital, a period of rehabilitation typically begins. This will generally involve short-term inpatient physical rehabilitation (rehab), such as at a skilled nursing or rehab facility. This initial focus of rehab is getting your physical strength back and regaining normal activities of daily living. It may also involve a period of time living in a supervised setting, especially for patients who live alone.

6.1. Physical Therapy

Physical therapy will play a cornerstone in regaining strength and mobility back after aneurysm clipping surgery. Generally, to achieve the highest level of progress, your physical therapist will utilize a wide range of exercise equipment in addition to their skills in planning the best recovery path for each individual patient. The ability of the exercises to work and the probabilities of their implementation will be related to a group of variables such as the area where the aneurysm ruptured, the age and general physical condition of the patient, the general patient's clinical condition, the level of initial disability, and the time passed from the intervention. A different recovery path will also be established from case to case. The professional present at your side will be able to return fundamental abilities to play sports and carry out everyday activities with an approach that includes a sequence of initial treatment, then the progressive use of exercise equipment, until the final result will be the use of equipment to strengthen methods of physical re-education alongside the professional, which will aid those who want to practice these sports, and in the most serious cases, to return running once more.

During physical therapy treatment after brain clipping surgery, common exercises and interventions that may be implemented to help restore function include aerobic capacity exercises and musculoskeletal strengthening. A physical therapy program may be tailored to the patient's individual tolerance and specific areas of physical deficiencies. It is important to target weak areas to restore the ability to carry out essential activities of daily living (ADL) as much as possible. The focus of physical therapy after a hemorrhagic stroke and aneurysm clipping is to work on strategies to maximize function within the patient's new level of ability. Clinicians aim to teach patients to integrate the weak side of the body when performing tasks.

Comprehensive Guide to Brain Aneurysm Clipping Surgery

1. Introduction to Brain Aneurysms

Furthermore, there are various types of brain aneurysms based on their location in the brain and how they are formed. Our series offers an in-depth exploration of brain aneurysms, brain aneurysm procedures, treatment possibilities, what to ask the medical team, and some personal stories of people who have lived through brain aneurysms with the guidance of our group of skilled the Johns Hopkins team physicians. When you're ready to study a lot more about surgery for brain aneurysms, continue reading our post on brain aneurysm clippings.

If you or someone you know has been diagnosed with a brain aneurysm, you may have begun examining potential treatment options. If you need more details about how to fix a brain aneurysm, it is also helpful to comprehend what, at its most simple level, the term really denotes. A brain aneurysm is characterized as a bulge in the blood vessel wall, or an artery, that supplies oxygenated blood to an area in the brain. Because there is little brain capacity to buffer high-pressure blood, brain aneurysm walls are commonly weak. Individuals with brain aneurysms are frequently diagnosed with a brain hemorrhage (subarachnoid hemorrhage), which occurs when the weak brain aneurysm bursts.

1.1. Definition and Types of Brain Aneurysms

There are two types of aneurysms in the brain, and they are as follows: 1. Saccular Aneurysms: This type of aneurysm is known to be the most common type and is shaped like a berry. According to research, saccular aneurysm occurs between the age of 35 to 60. These aneurysms are mostly located at the base of the arteries in the brain but can develop anywhere artery exists in the brain. 2. Mycotic: This type of aneurysm occurs as a result of bacterial or fungal infection which travels through the blood and causes the weakening of the arteries in the brain. Familial aneurysms and multiple aneurysms are other types of aneurysm. In 85% of the aneurysms that occur, there is no familial history of the aneurysm while in 15% of the patients who have this condition are as a result of having at least one family that has a brain aneurysm. Many of the brain aneurysm conditions are closed and do not heal while 10% of them break and bring about hemorrhagic strikes. The Doppler scans are used to diagnose brain aneurysms by professionals.

Aneurysms refer to weak areas present in the arteries of the brain tissue where there is protrusion of the arterial wall. Aneurysms commonly develop in the arteries located at the base of the brain. Glass primer used a grading scale for categorizing a ruptured brain aneurysm based on the severity of the bleeding which ranges from zero to 5.

1.2. Risk Factors and Symptoms

Symptoms: Symptoms can occur suddenly or at any time. Symptoms are sudden and severe headaches, stiff neck, seizures, rapid shortness of breath, nausea and vomiting, doubled or blurred vision, imbalance, sensitivity to light, or stroke-like symptoms. Brain aneurysms are often found during imaging tests for another reason if they show no symptoms at all. From diagnostic tests for other diseases, they've turned up, such as an MRI or CT scan. But you have an unruptured brain aneurysm if you experience some signs and symptoms of a ruptured or leaky aneurysm or if the aneurysm is large and has not yet ruptured, you will need to explore treatment choices. It depends on several factors, such as the position, shape, size and overall condition of your aneurysm. For some people with an aneurysm, another operation called an aneurysm-clipping.

Risk factors: People who have one or more of the following factors are more likely to develop a brain aneurysm: family history of brain aneurysms, are older, have certain inherited disorders, smoke, abuse drugs, high blood pressure, infections, blood disorders, and radiation. People who have one of the symptoms above are at a higher risk of developing a ruptured brain aneurysm.

2. Understanding Brain Aneurysm Clipping Surgery

An aneurysm whose root is bared to the blood flow escaping through it can be clipped to keep blood from inflating the aneurysm. Brain aneurysm clipping surgery requires the patient to be admitted to the hospital and undergo a two-hour or more surgical plan. An aneurysm entails an ongoing risk of rupture resulting in hemorrhage. An untreated aneurysm can rupture again or continue to grow and put a person at a higher risk of bleeding. Hurried surgery, such as a burst aneurysm, can have more difficulties than planned surgery. Brain aneurysm clipping is a surgical treatment for the removal of a ballooned area of a bursting or maintained blood vessel in the brain. During this surgery, a neurosurgeon will cut open the skull, and then use a microscope to locate and place a tiny clip across the neck of the aneurysm, allowing blood to shift normally round it. It avoids further bleeding for most aneurysms to be cut off. Brain aneurysms are often repaired using microsurgical strategies. This is performed with a microscope, surgical tools, and a microscope endoscope for an in-depth view.

A brain aneurysm refers to a bulge or ballooning in a blood vessel in the brain. Many aneurysms cause no symptoms or signs and may only be mentioned during tests for other conditions. Untreated aneurysms can crack or burst. When an aneurysm cracks or bursts, it can cause bleeding in the brain, often referred to as a hemorrhagic stroke.

Depending on the location, size, and shape, some aneurysms can break over time, and some are at higher risk of bursting than others. In cerebral aneurysm treatment, the aim is to keep the aneurysm from bursting or assist in treating it if already ruptured.

2.1. Purpose and Benefits

A brain aneurysm clipping surgery will have the best potential benefits for those who: have precise features within the aneurysm, like a lengthy slender channel, but without the branches; can tolerate the possible risks associated with surgery; are in good general health.

This is the most common primary operative method to cure a brain aneurysm, which involves a detailed and magnified view of the existing aneurysm and then placing a tiny metal clip across the sagging section of a weak artery (aneurysm). This surgery securely confines blood movement into the brain aneurysm and thereby effectively prevents stroke and death risks caused by a ruptured brain aneurysm. When the leakage is ceased from the aneurysm, the aneurysm will ultimately fade away over time.

As a solution to brain aneurysm that cannot be cured through blood pressure medication, brain aneurysm clipping surgery has become popular for brain aneurysms that feature a relatively safe dome and delicate branches. Thus, it is critical to recognize what type of brain aneurysm requires surgery, and in this section, we provide an exhaustive review of various relevant aspects of brain aneurysm surgery to educate the healthcare practitioners and public to assist in choosing the most appropriate treatment.

2.2. Comparison with Other Treatment Options

Clipping from clipping to coiling continues to be the primary hospital once it comes to aneurysm treatment for brain aneurysms. An aneurysm clip made of titanium or other form of material is bound to a piece of skull with opening. We used open brain surgery. After the metal clip is positioned surrounding the aneurysm mouth and then cut off the blood cell, the blood source to the nurture is prevented. This avoids rupture or flow back into the brain sanctuary. Some aneurysm clippings can also be completed with a stereotactic system. Coaching is performed as through endovascular form of procedure to coil. The coil is passed through a detachable stent through the groin or the arm in the aneurysm until the blood source to the wall is humiliated and push to our treatment area at the end of an aneurysm is finished. This prevents bleeding or flow back into the brain.

Clipping vs. Coiling:

A coiling procedure is a non-surgical variety of endovascular therapy. In the aneurysm, a wire loop is twisted. A stent-assisted coiling procedure implantation may prevent coil particles from leaving the aneurysm. A whole flow of the blood is halted after stent coiling is performed. Either procedure requires a wound in the groin or arm to be run through by a catheter.

Endovascular Treatment Options:

Compared to other available therapies:

What are the major differences of this surgery compared to other therapies that are available on the market? With this treatment choice, is it possible to avoid surgery and find a solution for the health problem? Have a look at some of the key techniques in brain aneurysm treatment below.

3. Preparation for Surgery

Surgical anesthesia is usually divided into two methods; first is a general anesthesia and the second is local anesthesia. Although it has its pros and cons, the decision as to which type of anesthesia will be administered depends on the anesthetist who adjusted to the conditions of each patient. On general anesthesia, the patient will be asleep which requires that they do not eat or drink 6 hours before surgery. This experience can be seen less favorable than local anesthesia, which has the advantage of reducing long-term complications after the surgery. For people who will carry out surgery, the first step that needs to be done before surgery is to fast at least 6 hours. If not done, it is the possibility of vomiting and vomited into his mouth, which in turn could go into the respiratory tract. In addition to fasting, the doctor adjusting medicines that are taken in advance, particularly with respect to diabetes. That is, during the treatment period, the patient should not take any medication. Thus, without the supervision adjustment, surgery will be canceled. And for women, it is recommended to remove the nail or toenail that has been applied in advance. The reason is that a blood vessel in the hands and feet is the first place the anesthesia given to the patient. In this case, the surgical dressings are clean is a very important thing, in fact, very vital. If the surgical openings arrive dirty, it will make no small risk of infection. In connection with this, before the surgery, the doctor WFA at least twice in washing his hands and wrists. At the end of 1990, a new hospital surgery has identified an effective mouthwash in the prevention of SSI (surgical site infection) are. Recent studies show controversy about chlorhexidine, a chemical used as a mouthwash that serves as an antiseptic. The report by Nagar et al (2007) mentions the use of 10-15 ml of a mouthwash containing alcohol and chlorhexidine. Half an hour before the operation begins. The second use antiseptic solutions, and that includes even an alcohol-based solution. This sterilization solution can remove all the microorganisms gathered in the skin or soft tissue surrounding the incision.

Before undergoing brain aneurysm clipping surgery, the patient has to prepare for it ahead of time to ensure that everything beforehand is in order. In the pre-surgery phase, the surgeon will usually send the patient to do a new diagnostic test such as MRI, CTA, MRA, and Digital Subtraction Angiography as the previous one has to be done prior to the first surgery or the surgery is no longer than 3 months of the previous test. Past 3 months, the patient has to undergo the test again. There are several things that underwent diagnostic tests such as CTA, MRA, and Digital Subtraction Angiography. First is that contrast may be inserted when the doctor needs it. Second is that it serves as a marker for surgical incision. Third is to facilitate the surgical procedure. Another thing for those who live outside of the area, it is enough for a visit at least three days before the operation is done after the test is performed. Patients do not need to be admitted to the hospital right away after the examination of shunting. Those who live in Eastern Indonesia, it should visit at least

4 days before the shunt test is done. Patients who live in the area close enough, stay 1-3 days expected after the drainage test is done.

3.1. Diagnostic Tests

This test can show stroke, injury, or malfunction. It's also utilized to pick the right treatment or check how well your brain aneurysm repair is going. In a CT angiography (CTA), a doctor inserts a special dye into a vein in your arm. This allows them to see your brain's blood vessels on an X-ray. In preparation for the procedure and during surgery, the anesthesiologist and your physician will ask you many questions about your medical history, medications, and allergies. Tell your doctor if you take any drugs regularly, drink alcohol, or use illicit drugs. Anticoagulants (blood thinners) or aspirin medications should be stopped 7 to 14 days before certain procedures. Your doctor will ask you to stop taking these medications if at all possible. Based on his or her expert judgment, the surgeon will adjust the discontinuation time accordingly. It's crucial that you notify your surgeon and anesthesiologist of all medications, including nonprescription drugs, herbal supplements, or other drugs. It is also important to follow directions for preoperative showers, eating and drinking, and medications. Your healthcare provider may order additional medical evaluations before surgery, including lab testing to check your kidney function or a urine test.

Before your operation, your physician will order special tests to determine the size, shape, and location of an aneurysm. Some of these tests may already be completed. Your medical records will be reviewed by your physician. You may need blood work and a urinalysis. Urinalysis is a laboratory test that examines urine. This test is used to screen for kidney or gallbladder disease, as well as diabetes. The following tests may be recommended by your surgeon to help prepare for your surgical procedure: Computed tomography (CT) scan and Magnetic resonance imaging (MRI), Angiography (arteriography), Blood Tests, Urinalysis, Chest X-Ray, and Electrocardiogram (ECG).

3.2. Medication and Lifestyle Adjustments

If possible, begin lowering your risk for stroke and other health problems that may occur. An enlarged or burst brain aneurysm can occur at the same time as a stroke, and some problems have overlapping risk factors. Likewise, a SAH due to a burst brain aneurysm may stimulate a stroke system. If you develop a brain aneurysm, even if it's only a sac and hasn't burst yet, you can take strides to avoid a rupture or discomfort due to a leaky aneurysm. Eating healthy, exercising, and not smoking are all beneficial. In cases when you don't require brain aneurysm repair, it's even more crucial to reduce potentially controllable stroke risk factors.

Once doctors have diagnosed you with a brain aneurysm, they will start preparing you for brain aneurysm clipping surgery. Some of the changes you make in your medications and lifestyle will only be temporary, while others may be permanent. You should take all medications your doctor prescribes as directed, and always consult with your doctor before stopping. Be sure to tell your doctor about all therapeutic and non-therapeutic drugs you're taking. Part of preparation for brain aneurysm clipping surgery includes modifying medications and lifestyle as you get ready for your operation. This will help minimize your risk of side effects during surgery. Your doctor may also decide to begin a medication that will help keep your aneurysm in check until your surgery date. These medications may also relieve symptoms before the surgery.

4. The Surgical Procedure

Clipping technique Clipping is often performed under the operating microscope. The surgeon locates the aneurysm, surrounding arteries, and any nearby important brain structures. Scopes may be used to assist in the exposure and treatment paths. A temporary clip is placed on the artery which goes into the aneurysm. A special type of clip is then placed across the bottom of the aneurysm after which the temporary clip is removed. The two clips create a "surgical block" to trap the aneurysm and prevent it from re-bleeding. It is important not to break the aneurysm when placing the two clips. Tissues are checked carefully for remaining hidden (in and under) the aneurysm in case surgical clips cannot control the aneurysm and the deep aneurysm bleeding occurs. Surgeons often have to use permanent clips and digital measurement tools under microscopes.

Incision A curved incision - 3 to 5 inches in length - is made behind the hairline. While making the incision, the hair in the surgical area is shaved or clipped. The surgery takes place under a high-power-operating microscope. A hole (craniotomy) is made by removing bone to allow access to the aneurysm and to decrease pressure on the brain. Muscle layers and other structures lining the skull are then spread apart to make a path to the aneurysm. Occasionally, muscle or a small piece of the sinus lining may need to be detached from the bone. The plastic or metal hair clips are placed around the hairline to help hold the skin edges together or to assist in returning a displaced hairline to its normal location.

Anesthesia Patients are put to sleep (general anesthesia) for microsurgery. Monitoring, including EEG, intracranial pressure, and drained fluid output, is used during the surgery. The anesthesia equipment is placed on the surgical side of the patient's head. X-rays are used to ensure that the patient is positioned properly.

The basic steps of the surgical procedures are similar, regardless of where or by whom they are performed.

4.1. Anesthesia and Incision

A coronal skin flap is raised, just behind the hairline, to require a curvilinear or linear incision that can be tailored to involve areas of hair growth in those with cosmetic concerns. In cases of long, transverse incisions, it is best to choose the 'beauty temporadalis' incision located behind the hairline in the 'beauty crease,' which involves a cosmetic incision with minimal alopecia. The skin flap is raised in a subperiosteal plane to avoid skin necrosis. A horseshoe-shaped periosteal flap is reflected superiorly, providing exposure to the anterior cranial vault and inferiorly serving the A1 segment of the anterior cerebral artery. The craniotomy performed is dependent on aneurysm location. Prior to performing the craniotomy, the head should be rotated towards the side of the aneurysm to determine the location of the midpupillary line. To aid in better visualization, a three-pin-horseshoe head clamp is applied to the head of the patient. The craniotomy is customized specifically for the aneurysm location in each patient and will be chosen on a case-per-case basis.

Incision:

Oxygen as an anesthetic has been the paradigm of anesthesia for intracranial craniotomy until newer developments with inhaled or other intravenous agents. Remifentanil, an ultrashort-acting synthetic opioid, was also found useful. General anesthetic agents should be administered with caution as they may cause increased intracranial pressure. Neurogenic pulmonary edema can occur from clipping of coiled large aneurysms; neurogenic pulmonary edema is believed to be mediated by the activity of sympathetic noradrenergic overactivity. Ultrashort-acting agents like remifentanil, atracurium are generally recommended for muscle relaxation. In certain aneurysm locations, positioning the patient can also present a lot of technical difficulties; ideally, the head needs to be positioned in such a way to aid in reducing brain retraction. Keeping the head of the bed slightly elevated helps to aid in better venous drainage and decreases blood in the operative field.

Anesthesia:

4.2. Clipping Technique and Tools

Several clips may be placed on the aneurysm until no blood flows through it. In addition, sometimes, post-clipping catheter angiograms are performed to make sure there are no clips that are too tight and causing problems downstream. Special heating tools may also be used during surgery to help the blood vessels heal around the clip to create a secure closure.

Clipping a brain aneurysm involves cutting a window into the skull and working around the brain to place the clip. Often, a portion of your skull will be temporarily removed and replaced using titanium plates and screws. The incision in the skin is then closed using stitches or staples. Newer suture methods are used to avoid leaving a depressed area on the skull where the surgery was performed. Sometimes, dissolvable sutures are used on the skin to avoid the need for a second surgery to remove stitches or staples. The tools used to open the skull and perform brain aneurysm clipping surgery include motorized drills, bone flaps, dilators, dissecting tools, and micro neurosurgical techniques that require a microscope.

The technique used to clip a brain aneurysm depends on the direction of the aneurysm, its size and location, and the blood vessels around it. Temporary clipping is sometimes used to help surgeons determine how to properly place the clipped aneurysm. Once the aneurysm has been removed from the normal blood flow, the clip holds the edges of the opening in the blood vessel closed, preventing the aneurysm from refilling with blood.

5. Recovery and Rehabilitation

In the majority of situations, you will most likely be required to engage in physical therapy to supplement your rehabilitation process. An occupational therapist is a professional who assists people in relearning fundamental daily activities such as eating, going to the bathroom, and bathing. If your aneurysm has formed in areas of the brain that control speech or language, speech and language therapy is an additional sort of cognitive therapy that your physician might suggest. Furthermore, many individuals who have undergone clipping surgery may have debilitated short-term memory or cognitive deficits, which can be improved with the assistance of cognitive therapy. For body weight, high blood pressure, asthma, and other chronic health issues, your doctor may change your medications. It is possible that you'll be prescribed new medications as well.

During your stay in the hospital, you will have frequent check-ups to ensure that your progress is favorable and that you are not experiencing severe complications that would require attention. About seven to ten days following the operation, most patients are able to journey home. In order to allow the surgical site to properly heal, you will need roughly two to four weeks to rest at home following your discharge from the hospital. Once you are home, on your caregiver's aid and upon your physician's approval, avoid the usage of any medicines that contain Ibuprofen or Aspirin.

Following brain aneurysm clipping surgery, most patients will need to recover in an intensive care unit for a day or two before being transferred to a hospital room. This breathtaking procedure usually takes anywhere from three to five hours to complete, but it could run longer in more challenging cases. You may experience the effects of the procedure for one or more days following surgery, such as mood changes and trouble focusing.

5.1. Postoperative Care

Gradually, the nursing staff will work to wake the patient up more. Incidentally, your head may be wrapped to protect the wound, and sutures close up the operative area. Once stable, patients will return to their hospital room. The temporary postoperative period has further precautions that need to be adhered to: the patient will be instructed to avoid straining (such as pushing, lifting, coughing, and using the bathroom), avoid laying flat, stretching your neck, hanging it over the bed, or straining to look upwards, adhere to activity restrictions until later instructed, and call for assistance to move and do things, including using the bathroom or bath, until they are cleared otherwise.

Postoperative care after surgery is critical when the patient awakens from anesthesia. Once the surgery is over, the patient is transferred to the recovery room. As the patient wakes up from anesthesia, the nurse monitors the patient's vital signs while the patient rests in a semi-upright position. This position allows for reduced blood circulation to the operative site. It is unusual for the patient to wake up with a clear head right away; many patients go on to intensive care or another similar area.

5.2. Physical and Cognitive Therapy

Cognitive treatment primarily focuses on language and understanding issues as well as comprehensive structure problems that also arise as side effects following brain aneurysm pruning. It is important for patients to get a speech and language review while they are in the hospital so that customized speech and speech pathology care can be established. All patients would have different speech and experience learning limitations, and cognitive treatment should be very appealing to this individual patient.

Physical therapy, as a common treatment method, primarily aims at helping the body rebuild its energy, stamina, versatility, stability, coordination, and the proper handling of pain. When post-surgery pain is kept under control, it becomes very valuable for patients to maintain building up nap muscles along with aerobic energy. Posture rehabilitation is also another helpful component in the lifespan after craniotomy. Learning how to stand, walk, build weight on spare helping ears or limbs, flexing the neck to compel optimal walking or sitting alignments is critical. Electrical stimulation for gait and gluteals (familiar to the body through the use of another name EMS) is also utilized for craniotomy patients to rehabilitate. I think physical treatment is also necessary to get the craniotomy stitches or strips changed and assist with outpatient office visits.

When it comes to pruning an aneurysm of the brain, the majority of patients will tell you that cognitive and physical therapies have a larger impact on their recovery process. It is beneficial to have a deeper understanding of the role any of these treatments will play in successfully welcoming someone's livelihood.

6. Risks and Complications

Your neurosurgeon will speak with you and your caregivers before the aneurysm surgery day in detail about what potential complications they may anticipate for the aneurysm itself, as well as those stemming from the surgery.

- Short-term problems with thinking or processing information, because the brain is likely to be swollen during the recovery period - Trouble with balance - Seizures - Headaches - Hydrocephalus, which can take a while to develop and may require additional treatment with shunt surgery - Re-bleeding if the aneurysm is only partially blocked off or if the treated aneurysm is especially large or complex - Stroke due to a blood clot that developed on a blood vessel in response to the presence of the aneurysm or sales packs placed in the brain tissue

Even after you leave the hospital and recover from surgery, there are still some potential long-term complications of having brain aneurysm clipping surgery. Some of these include:

- Brain swelling - Bleeding into the brain - Vasospasm (when a blood vessel constricts, reducing the amount of blood that can flow through it) - Hydrocephalus (when there is an accumulation of cerebrospinal fluid inside the brain) - The aneurysm rupturing during surgery or afterward - Stroke or a stroke-like event - Infection - Air embolism, a rare but potentially serious complication that can occur if a blood vessel used during surgery leaks air - Complications due to the use of medications or other anesthetics

Some of the most common early surgery complications include:

Like all surgeries, there are risks involved with the brain aneurysm clipping procedure. Temporary or permanent complications can occur both during surgery and within the recovery time immediately afterward, or can be seen longer term beyond the recovery period.

6.1. Immediate Risks

Morbidity, if survived, is certain. Major disability is often present to varying degrees with almost all patients. The various dialogs necessitated to define these outcomes prior to treatment are established to be very important for effective discussions with families. The mortality of brain aneurysm clipping surgery is greatest in patients with SAH+. There are immediate risks that all brain aneurysm surgery patients face. These immediate risks may lead to cerebral ischemia or infarction, arrhythmia, seizure, paralysis, cognitive deficits, aphasia, cranial nerve deficits, numbness, facial weakness, coma, vegetative state, brain death, and hydrocephalus. There are also a variety of potential reactions caused by brain anesthesia such as pneumonia, urinary tract infections, and electrolyte disturbances in the brain. Post clipping BP variability of systolic BP ± 20mmHg has no significance in TCDs vasospasm screening prediction.

Ischemic stroke or transient ischemic attack refers to a blockage in an artery that reduces blood flow to the brain. As the brain relies on a constant supply of oxygen and nutrients, when this is cut off, it can lead to irreversible damage. The sudden and chronic loss of consciousness often occurs amid an ischemic event and may never return. Rerupture of the aneurysm is the collection of blood inside the skull resulting from spontaneous and premature post-surgical opening of the aneurysm. When adding the added volume of the blood from the debrided aneurysm to the original neurologic injury of the aneurysm rupture, that

can all result in subsequent permanent brain damage or
death.

6.2. Long-Term Considerations

Blood Vessel Anxiety of Angiogram Remifentanil (BVAAR) is when a person feels anxious, stressed, overwhelmed, fearful, or panicked as they prepare for an angiogram, during the angiogram procedure, waiting for an angiogram to be performed, and/or at the time of the angiogram being performed. This may be due to the anxiety around the procedure, the visit to the center, the hospital setting, the feelings, the thoughts, the treatment, and/or the multiple people involved at the center. This may result in physical side effects. Brain surgery depends on the area of the brain the aneurysm is located, its size, and if the patient suffers from any other medical problems. Aneurysm surgery (clipping), post-surgery considerations: patients who have clipping surgery for brain aneurysms are typically in the hospital 4-7 days, going home when they are healthy.

Though post-surgery symptoms will likely dissipate within a few months, and maybe within a few weeks, other symptoms and cognitive difficulties can last for years. Much of this has to do with the placement of the clip and any damage that was done to the brain from the bleeding aneurysm. Many survivors of clipping surgery do heal and can expect to live normal lives within a couple of years after surgery. It is important to keep that in mind when you are faced with difficulties. We hope this information gives you an idea of what to expect and, at the very least, brings validation to what you may be experiencing. Long-term complications also include blood flow changes, cognitive and speech issues, headaches, hydrocephalus, medialization, memory loss, psychological changes, and seizures.

7. Outcomes and Prognosis

There are also individual-related factors that can influence outcome following brain aneurysm clipping surgery. An individual's overall health can play a role in the potential occurrence of complications after surgery and in how fast they recover. In addition, there are published prognostic prediction models which can estimate the chances of severe physical disability or death for an individual over the long-term. These models analyze various patient characteristics to make these longer-term predictions, including aspects of the initial aSAH presentation as well as the general health of a patient at the time of rupture. Certain aspects of brain MRI, such as the appearance of the cisterns, have also been linked to prognosis following brain aneurysm surgery. Ultimately, prognosis is something that can be highly variable between individuals. Post-surgery, compliance with long-term medical care and monitoring can play an important role in the prevention of future bleeding, aneurysm regrowth or new aneurysm development, and management of other medical problems.

Brain aneurysm clipping surgery is a commonly performed procedure with a high success rate. A large majority of patients who undergo clipping experience no complications from the surgery. For some patients, residual symptoms may persist even after the aneurysm is blocked, but post-surgery rehab and management can help address them. Patients may also experience a recurrence of bleeding over time. This occurs in less than 1 out of 20 patients who undergo surgical clipping and typically results from a new aneurysm that develops rather than from weakened incisions or from an aneurysm gradually reforming. Outcomes from aneurysmal subarachnoid hemorrhage may depend on various factors. Generally speaking, patients who experience aSAH from a brain aneurysm do better following an ultimate outcome the longer they go without another bleed. Treatment with clipping or coiling generally improves aSAH prognosis compared to no treatment. Fittingly, when present, the recommendations for most patients who carry an unruptured brain aneurysm at diagnosis is to undergo clipping or coiling to prevent a rupture from occurring in the future.

7.1. Success Rates and Factors Affecting Prognosis

Head imaging – Any condition or diagnosis captured in the imaging results of the head following a scan could alter the prediction of the worst position. It is also important for you to discuss this finding with your doctor.

Patient – Size, shape, location, and patient's type of aneurysm - Some types of aneurysms are technically more difficult to repair than others. More complex surgeries may lead to slightly reduced success rates. On the contrary, standard aneurysms and simple surgeries are more trustworthy - whether or not the aneurysm or an easy-to-access artery.

Though prognosis is highly individualized and depends on numerous patient factors, experts have identified a few key factors that can play a role in determining how well a patient does after treatment for aneurysm. It is important to review with your surgeon.

Factors affecting prognosis (likely outcome)

b. The success rate also decreases if the ruptured aneurysm is significant, allowing large blood flow to the brain and putting pressure on surrounding tissues. Presence of hematoma also lowers the prognosis. In other words, surgery on atypical ruptured aneurysm is less certain than treatment on a repetitive aneurysm.

a. In the case of new, recent, or ruptured aneurysm, the success rate is lower than the success rate of 97% to 98%

(as in the case of non-ruptured aneurysm). Largely, patients with broken aneurysm who get the treatment instantly have an extremely high success rate of surgery.

It is tough to give a predictable or even approximate success rate for any surgical procedure, as numerous factors can play a role in its outcome. But generally, it can be said that most surgeries have a success rate of 90% or higher. The success rates of brain aneurysm clipping surgery are as follows:

Success rates in brain aneurysm clipping surgery

8. Research and Innovations

Because barbiturates and other medications are used to put patients to sleep for clipping, it may cause heavy sedation and induce sleep for a variable amount of time. Neurosurgeons must finish an undergraduate education and supplemental medical training to be entitled for certification. Besides being board-certified practicing neurosurgeons, all of our surgeons have extra years of fellowship training in the treatment of brain aneurysms. Our entire team is dedicated to making every effort to provide the most suitable and high-quality health care services to our patients and to make sure that the entire needs of patients are met while they are in our facility. Due to improvements in technology and microsurgery instruments, the size of the incision has dropped steadily and multiple culottes that are less invasive have been developed. We have received funds from the National Institute for Neurological Disabilities for aneurysm research using advancing technology, as well as from the Brain Aneurysm Foundation and many other grants.

Our caring support team offers important resources and services to guide you throughout the surgical clipping of an aneurysm, ensuring the best possible outcome. Our website provides a variety of resources that offer comprehensive details on our programs and services, answer commonly asked questions, and offer suggestions for your stay. The blood from these veins may be reabsorbed into the patient's system or occasionally a lumbar (spinal) drain is used to drain off this small accumulation of blood. You will be encouraged to determine the position of your hospital bed, if possible, in a raised position as long as it is comfortable for you.

8.1. Advancements in Surgical Techniques

Full Visualization Technique. Technological enhancement, including visualization devices for endoscopic-assisted microsurgery, aid complete visualization around target neurovascular structures. Microsurgical Clipping Without Preoperative Endovascular Therapy. Intraoperative monitoring, neuronavigation, Doppler flow ultrasound, and/or fluorescence apprise the surgeon about the neurovascular structures in proximity and/or within the field of microscopic operation. Cerebrospinal Fluid Diversion. This technical aspect was initially highlighted two decades ago. The authors have further emphasized the significance of cerebrospinal fluid (CSF) drainage for retraction of the cerebrum. The microsurgical corridors can be opened significantly by continuous CSF drainage. The expansion of the surgical anatomy space is limited in the subarachnoid space only. Hyperacute Surgery. Early surgery stands firm mainly on innovative clinical trial data and advanced intraoperative neurophysiological monitoring techniques.

Advancements in imaging, intraoperative neurophysiological monitoring, and microsurgical techniques now allow delicate dissection and precise proximal and/or distal clip placement at the neck of the aneurysm to be performed safely, thus reducing complications. Moreover, the recent advancements in neurosurgical knowledge and retraining of neurosurgeons have significantly improved the outcome of patients following brain aneurysm clipping. These skills require neurosurgeons to undergo consistent retraining. They must be able to handle delicate neurovasculature safely and expertly. Off late, additional interventional radiology procedures have been safely combined with surgical clipping to optimize the occlusion rate and minimize flow-related complications.

8.2. Clinical Trials and Future Directions

There are a few trials that show great promise. Some are
multi-disciplinary, but they remain imperative reading.
This includes the Barrow Ruptured Aneurysm Trial
(BRAT), which compares endovascular coiling to surgical
clipping. Initial results are anticipated soon. Regarding the
surgical treatment of unruptured cerebral aneurysms,
comparisons of rates of epilepsy in patients who have
aneurysms treated with endovascular therapy versus
microsurgical successful aneurysm clipping are being
studied in the prospective, randomized Barrow Treatment
of Unruptured Aneurysms Study (UNAT). The patients in
this study are randomly assigned by the surgeon to
clipping if the aneurysm topography is not amenable to
coiling or to crossing over to the primary coil treatment if
the aneurysm is not amenable to clipping. Each arm
includes 200 patients. Preliminary results are expected
soon.

It is surprisingly difficult to find high-quality, randomized
trial evidence related to surgical brain aneurysm
treatment. As the number of endovascular-brain aneurysm
treatments has climbed, fewer studies are published that
investigate microsurgical approaches to brain aneurysm
resection. In general, neurosurgeons have not had easy
access to funded trials from the government and industry
alike. Unfortunately, the vast majority of grants (for both
endovascular and microsurgery) are related to devices or
technology and not surgery itself. The National Institutes of
Health (NIH) and the Patient-Centered Outcomes Research

Institute (PCORI) are underutilized by neurosurgeons, and encouraging high quality and cost-efficient craniotomy and microsurgical brain aneurysm research opportunities remain underdeveloped.